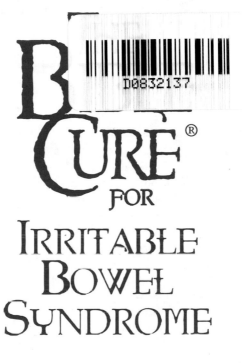

BIBLE CURE®

FOR

IRRITABLE BOWEL SYNDROME

DON COLBERT, M.D.

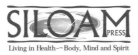

SILOAM PRESS

Living in Health—Body, Mind and Spirit

THE BIBLE CURE FOR IRRITABLE BOWEL SYNDROME
by Don Colbert, M.D.
Published by Siloam Press
A part of Strang Communications Company
600 Rinehart Road
Lake Mary, Florida 32746
www.siloampress.com

Library of Congress Cataloging Card Number: 2002101779
International Standard Book Number: 0-88419-827-8

This book is not intended to provide medical advice or to take the place of medical advice and treatment from your personal physician. Readers are advised to consult their own doctors or other qualified health professionals regarding the treatment of their medical problems. Neither the publisher nor the author takes any responsibility for any possible consequences from any treatment, action or application of medicine, supplement, herb or preparation to any person reading or following the information in this book. If readers are taking prescription medications, they should consult with their physicians and not take themselves off of medicines to start supplementation without the proper supervision of a physician.

02 03 04 05   8765432
Printed in the United States of America

Restoration Power
for You!

A unique characteristic of God's healing power in your life is His desire to renew and restore you—body, mind and spirit. The Bible says, "'I will restore you to health and I will heal you of your wounds,' declares the LORD" (Jer. 30:17, NAS).

As a matter of fact, restoration is a part of God's grand plan for everything and everyone on earth—including you! The Bible says, "Wonderful times of refreshment will come from the presence of the Lord, and he will send Jesus your Messiah to you again. For he must remain in heaven until the time for the final restoration of all things, as God promised long ago through his prophets" (Acts 3:20–21).

This promises that everything will be restored

in the right time, for restoration is at the heart of God's purpose and desire for you.

If you are suffering the symptoms of irritable bowel syndrome (IBS), then the chances are very good that you need a lot of restoration—of your body, mind and spirit. The roots of IBS are discovered in many factors of physical, mental and emotional depletion, including fatigue, chronic stress, long-term emotional turmoil and much more.

Addressing the Spiritual Roots of Disease

As a Christian medical doctor I've studied and prayed about the causes of disease for many years. Increasingly I've discovered that many diseases have very strong spiritual roots. If you are familiar with my books, then doubtless you are aware that I believe in the health of the entire person—body, mind and spirit. Although traditional medicine often sees these facets of our being as very separate, in truth they are not. A vital link exists between the spirit, soul and body. And although much of the disease and physical pain we suffer comes from the body, often these distresses begin in the spirit and the soul, which encompasses the mind and emotions.

Therefore, truly walking in the divine health that God intends for us at times requires that we look a little deeper, beyond the physical process of disease to the spiritual, mental and emotional roots. I trust that you will find these pages extremely enlightening as you gain new insight and revelation to help you live your life in the robust, joyful state of good health that God desires for you.

So, let's closely examine IBS—its roots, symptoms and characteristics—to gain some valuable, restorative insight into natural and biblical healing cures. Prepare to gain fresh insight and perspective into your disorder that can bring a new dimension of health, wholeness and refreshing to you.

The Secret's Out!

IBS, also known as spastic colon and nervous stomach, is the most common gastrointestinal disorder. One in five adults has some degree of it, which equals about thirty-five million people in the U.S. alone. Approximately twice as many women suffer from IBS as men, accounting for a whopping half of all visits to GI specialists and 10 percent of all family practitioner visits.

IBS is a *functional gastrointestinal disorder*, which means that its symptoms cannot be explained by any anatomical, physiological or biochemical abnormality. In other words, after performing a battery of tests including x-rays, blood tests and endoscopic exams of the GI tract, no biological cause for the symptoms can be found. Therefore, IBS is diagnosed from its symptoms, not by any medical exam or tests.

> *The Spirit of the Sovereign LORD is upon me, because the LORD has appointed me to bring good news to the poor. He has sent me to comfort the brokenhearted and to announce that captives will be released and prisoners will be freed. He has sent me to tell those who mourn that the time of the LORD's favor has come.*
> —ISAIAH 61:1–2

If you have IBS, your colon cannot always coordinate its function in a normal fashion; therefore, it spasms. It also tends to be more sensitive to certain food triggers and various dietary factors. In addition, your colon can be the location in your body where your emotional responses can be released through physical symptoms. In other words, your bowels can become a link between the spiritual conflict that you must daily battle, living in a pressure-cooker world—your level of stress—and your physical body.

In the Bible a man named Job suffered greatly during a particularly difficult season of trial. Job spoke about the effect his stressful situation was having upon his body. He lamented, "When I looked for good, then evil came unto me; and when I waited for light, there came darkness. My bowels boiled, and rested not: the days of affliction prevented me" (Job 30:26–27, KJV). Job's spiritual distress, by his own admission, caused great disturbance in his bowels. If you suffer with IBS, you already know what Job was talking about.

No matter what the root causes of your IBS, by picking up this Bible Cure booklet you have taken an exciting first step toward renewed health. With fresh wisdom about God's powerful principles of health and insight into God's power to heal, you can experience full restoration.

God revealed His divine will for you through the apostle John who wrote, "Dear friend, I am praying that all is well with you and that *your body is as healthy as I know your soul is*" (3 John 2, emphasis added).

This Bible Cure booklet is filled with hope and

encouragement for understanding how to keep your body fit and healthy. In this book, you will

uncover God's divine plan of health
for body, soul and spirit
through modern medicine,
good nutrition,
and the medicinal power of
Scripture and prayer.

You will find key scripture passages throughout this book that will help you focus on the power of God. These divine promises will empower your prayers and redirect your thoughts to line up with God's plan of divine health for you—a plan that includes victory over IBS and its destructive physical and spiritual roots.

In this Bible Cure booklet, you will gain a strategic plan for divine health in the following chapters:

If you are experiencing IBS, the chances are good that your body has been in a battle. Perhaps your mind and spirit have been, too. With fresh confidence and the dynamic knowledge that God is real, that He is alive and that He loves you more than you could ever imagine, you can enjoy complete restoration of your health—body, mind and spirit.

It is my prayer that these powerful godly insights will bring health, wholeness and spiritual refreshing to you—body, mind and spirit. May they deepen your fellowship with God and strengthen your ability to worship and serve Him.

—DON COLBERT, M.D.

Chapter 1

Refresh With Wisdom

A major purpose of God in your life is to refresh and renew your body, mind and spirit. The Bible says, "They that wait upon the LORD shall renew their strength; they shall mount up with wings as eagles; they shall run, and not be weary; and they shall walk, and not faint" (Isa. 40:31, KJV).

Gaining physical and spiritual refreshing and renewal require careful wisdom from God. Godly wisdom is a vital key to restoration for your body: "But the excellency of knowledge is, that wisdom giveth life to them that have it" (Eccles. 7:12, KJV).

A key reason for writing this Bible Cure booklet is to provide you with the wisdom you need to enjoy the health and strength of total renewal. And as I mentioned earlier, if you are suffering with IBS, then your body needs restoring. So, let's begin building a foundation of knowledge from which to gain dynamic wisdom to renew your health.

Six Telltale Symptoms

As previously mentioned, IBS is diagnosed by its symptoms. The six trademark symptoms of IBS are listed below. You will know you have IBS if you experience at least three of the six most common symptoms for over three months.

> *Don't worry about anything; instead, pray about everything. Tell God what you need, and thank him for all he has done. If you do this, you will experience God's peace, which is far more wonderful than the human mind can understand. His peace will guard your hearts and minds as you live in Christ Jesus.*
> —PHILIPPIANS 4:6–7

Abdominal pain

Have you been experiencing pain in your abdomen? If you have for more than three months, you may have IBS. This pain is the main symptom of IBS. It usually feels like a cramping pain, but it may be either sharp or dull. It is commonly located in the left lower quadrant of the abdomen. That's below the belly button and to the left. However, the pain can be felt throughout the entire abdomen. This pain usually is relieved by having a bowel movement or by passing gas.

Irregular bowel function

You may experience episodes of irregular bowel function, alternating with normal function. In other words, you may have either bouts of constipation or diarrhea, or both.

An urgency to have a bowel movement

An urgency to have a bowel movement that seemingly can strike at any time is another symptom. This urgency can be very unpredictable and very embarrassing. It will usually occur at meal times or shortly thereafter.

Abdominal swelling

Another very common symptom is abdominal swelling and bloating, which generally occurs after eating. The pain and swelling usually go away as you sleep.

Mucus in the stool

Mucus (without blood) in the stool is very common if you have IBS. Mucus is secreted by the lining of the colon and rectum, and it functions as a lubricant to ease the passage of the stool. If you have IBS, your body may produce extra mucus, but it is not dangerous and is not a sign of serious disease.

Incomplete emptying of the rectum

Another common symptom is a feeling of incomplete emptying of the rectum after a bowel movement. People suffering from IBS feel they have only had a partial bowel movement, and thus they strain more in an attempt to pass more stool. This is very hard on the anus and can lead to the development of hemorrhoids and eventually rectal prolapse (a condition that involves the lining of the rectum actually protruding from the body).

If you have at least three of these six symptoms for more than three months without symptoms of a bowel disease, you probably have IBS. Nevertheless, only your doctor can make a final determination. There is NO link between IBS and cancer.

> *I am leaving you with a gift—peace of mind and heart. And the peace I give isn't like the peace the world gives. So don't be troubled or afraid.*
> —John 14:27

However, if you are experiencing other painful symptoms, you may have an inflammatory bowel

4

disease such as Crohn's disease or ulcerative colitis. Approximately one million Americans have inflammatory bowel disease. Therefore, it's vitally important to get a correct diagnosis from your doctor. Consult your physician right away if you are experiencing the following symptoms, which could indicate a more serious condition:

- Blood in the stool
- Weight loss
- Fevers
- Waking up from sleep with bowel disturbances

A Closer Look

If your skin were to suddenly become completely transparent, this is what you'd see after eating. Your GI tract is similar to a thirty-foot-long tube that begins at your mouth and continues all the way to your anus.

The GI tract is much more complex than a tube. As a matter of fact, it is one of the most complex organ systems in your body. It has five main parts:

- Your mouth and pharynx
- Your esophagus (the tube that carries food from your mouth to your stomach)

- Your stomach
- Your small intestines
- Your colon (your large intestine up to your rectum and anus)

Following the Bagel Trail

Bite a bagel, and an amazing process begins that is completely hidden from sight. To better understand IBS, let's follow the bagel trail and see where it goes.

Take that bagel with cream cheese, and bite a big chunk out of it. Begin chewing, and the process of digestion is well under way. As you chew, you grind up the bagel, pulverizing it into very small particles so that it can be mixed with saliva, which is also a digestive juice.

> *When you go through deep waters and great trouble, I will be with you. When you go through rivers of difficulty, you will not drown! When you walk through the fire of oppression, you will not be burned up; the flames will not consume you.*
> —Isaiah 43:2

The bagel is swallowed and passes through your esophagus into your stomach so that it can continue being digested.

In the stomach, the bagel is churned around as if in a blender for about two hours. Hydrochloric acid and powerful digestive enzymes help to break the food down even more. When your bagel is finally ready to leave your stomach, it looks like thick soup that is referred to as *chyme*.

Very slowly your stomach empties its processed bagel into a one-inch diameter tube called the small intestine. The first section of the small intestine to receive the food is called the *duodenum*.

Your small intestine actually has three sections:

- The duodenum
- The jejunum
- The ileum

When your partially digested bagel reaches the duodenum, your pancreas releases even more enzymes to complete digestion. Your gallbladder also releases bile acids into the small intestine. These function like detergents, allowing the enzymes to mix thoroughly with the food contents.

All of this is taking place in the small intestine—a twenty-foot-long tube covered with millions of tiny fingerlike projections called *villi*. The villi absorb the processed nutrients into the bloodstream. If you spread out the surface area of the intestines and the villi, it would be approximately the surface area of a tennis court. Most of your food is absorbed in the second section of the intestine, the *jejunum*.

The third part of the small intestine is called the *ileum*. Here water is reabsorbed along with bile and other nutrients.

Continuing Along the Pathway

It takes about three to five hours for your bagel to make its way through the small intestine. From the small intestine, what's left dumps into the large intestine, which is primarily undigested food material.

The small intestine processes and reabsorbs a lot of fluids, such as saliva, stomach acid and pancreatic juices, along with bile from the gallbladder and other fluids that are actually secreted by the small intestine. Believe it or not, about eight to ten quarts of different digestive fluids are produced in your body each day. Most of these juices are reabsorbed in the ileum in the small intestine.

Passage Into the Colon

Most of the bagel's nutrients have been absorbed by the small intestine. The remains of the bagel, which is fiber and other unabsorbed material, continues on its path to the large intestine, also called the colon. It enters the colon from the small intestine through a valve called the *ileocecal valve.*

This vital valve allows undigested food material and unabsorbed fluid to be passed into the colon. Generally it takes about five hours for food that has been chewed in the mouth to reach the colon.

The Final Journey

Once undigested food material reaches the colon, it usually takes another one to two full days of processing in the colon before it's eliminated in the stool. A high-fiber diet would shorten its stay in the colon.

Every day approximately 1 to 1½ quarts of fluid and liquefied food enter the colon through the ileocecal valve. At this point, much of your bagel has already been processed and is well

> *And this same God who takes care of me will supply all your needs from his glorious riches, which have been given to us in Christ Jesus.*
> —PHILIPPIANS 4:19

on its way to your bloodstream, energizing your organs, muscles and other tissues with vitamins, minerals and glucose for fuel.

This large intestine is about five feet long and about two and a half inches wide. Once inside the colon, the remains of your bagel meet up with about four hundred different kinds of bacterial microorganisms that weigh about 3 pounds Some of this bacteria is beneficial for you, and some of it is not. If your body is in relatively good health, then the good bacteria will outnumber the nonbeneficial bacteria.

These friendly bacteria break down some of the undigested food material and fiber.

Move It Along

How does the food and liquid move through the large intestine? It is propelled through the hollow tube by wavelike contractions called *peristalsis*. The solid mass of undigested food is moved by these waves from the right side of your body to the left where it will eventually be eliminated from the rectum.

Peristalsis usually occurs in a regular and rhythmic pattern of contraction and relaxation. Pain commonly occurs when the contractions increase. Eating a meal usually causes the contractions to increase; this is called the *gastrocolic reflex*. This reflex enables the colon and rectum to eliminate stool as new food is starting to enter the stomach. Many individuals with IBS have a hyperactive gastrocolic reflex, which may cause diarrhea and pain after eating.

When the stool finally enters the rectum, the stretching of the rectum causes the muscles in the rectum and anus to relax so that the stool can be eliminated. Glands in the colon produce mucus to coat the stool, thus allowing for easier passage.

What Causes It?

Irritable bowel syndrome may be related to other intestinal assaults, such as food poisoning or gastroenteritis. We will discuss briefly some common causes of IBS.

The Fury of Food Poisoning

An infection of the intestinal tract known as *gastroenteritis* can cause IBS. Salmonella, a species of pathogenic bacteria, is often the culprit. Infections are usually caused by improperly preparing and cooking chicken, eggs and other meats. It's possible to mistake mild cases of food poisoning with the flu and not even realize that you had it. Although this food poisoning is usually mild, in some rare instances it can be fatal.

Bacterial assaults are not the only cause for IBS.

Painful Problems With Parasites

Parasites and viruses can cause IBS, too. If you think that the only folks who get parasites are those who travel and live in poor Third World countries, you are mistaken. As a matter of fact, you may have parasites living in your body right now!

Intestinal parasites are either protozoa, which are one-celled organisms, or worms, such as tapeworms or roundworms. They live off a host (you) and can cause a lot of damage to your GI tract. Parasitic infections are a lot more common

> *Fix your thoughts on what is true and honorable and right. Think about things that are pure and lovely and admirable. Think about things that are excellent and worthy of praise.*
> —Philippians 4:8

here in the United States than most people think. In fact, more than 130 species of intestinal parasites are found in North America. Most of the world's population is colonized by them. You've probably been among them, and you may even have them right now.

Parasites can cause gastroenteritis with diarrhea and intestinal damage that can persist for months, even after you've been treated for the parasite attack.

Fortunately, the irritable bowel syndrome that develops after parasitic gastroenteritis usually only lasts for a few weeks. However, it can last for months or even years after a severe bout of parasitic gastroenteritis.

Love Milk—but It Doesn't Love You?

Lactose intolerance is an inability to properly digest milk and milk products. Its symptoms are very similar to irritable bowel syndrome, even though it is classified as a separate condition.

If you are experiencing lactose intolerance, your symptoms may include any or all of the following: diarrhea, bloating, gas and abdominal cramps.

During digestion lactose, or milk sugar, is normally broken down into simple sugars called monosaccharides, glucose and galactose. To do this effectively, your body needs the enzyme *lactase*.

If you don't have enough lactase in your body, lactose remains in your GI tract causing diarrhea, bloating, gas and abdominal cramps.

If you are lactose intolerant, you're certainly not alone. Your ethnic origins play a major role in determining whether or not you are lactose intolerant. About 20 percent of Caucasians, 75 percent of African Americans and an amazing 80 percent of Asian Americans are lactose intolerant. About half of Hispanic Americans are lactose intolerant.

For the lactose intolerant, about two hours after drinking milk or eating ice cream, soft cheeses and other dairy products, the uncomfortable symptoms will start.

Antibiotic Attacks on the Gut

Although antibiotics are modern wonders that have helped many individuals, they can be quite harmful if used too often or for too long a period of time.

Using antibiotics over an extended period of time can lead to IBS. Using powerful antibiotics, even for a short duration, can trigger irritable bowel syndrome in some individuals.

Some doctors use antibiotics recurrently or for a prolonged period of time to treat infections such as acne, chronic sinusitis, sore throats, ear infections, recurrent bronchitis, pneumonia, prostatitis and other infections. Although antibiotics aggressively attack infections, they can also wreak havoc on your intestinal flora (or the delicate balance of good bacteria). That's because antibiotics don't just kill the bad bacteria. They kill all bacteria, both good and bad.

The antibiotics taken to cure infections can actually cause an infection in the colon. An example of this is *pseudomembranous colitis,* caused by the bacterium *Clostridium difficile.* In other words, antibiotic use can actually lead to a more dangerous infection of the colon.

In addition, overuse of antibiotics can lead to bacterial overgrowth in the small intestine. Although bacteria normally thrive in your healthy colon, they should not grow in your small intestine. When bacteria grow out of control and begin inhabiting your small intestine, they start to compete with you for nutrition. Once inside the

> *Those who live in the shelter of the Most High will find rest in the shadow of the Almighty. This I declare of the LORD: He alone is my refuge, my place of safety; he is my God, and I am trusting him.*
> —PSALM 91:1–2

small intestine, these bacteria ferment carbohy-drates and starches and produce excessive gas, bloating and abdominal pain.

Candida Calamities

Along with the colonies of bacteria inside your colon is yeast, or candida. It is usually quite normal and harmless because its growth is held in check by the good bacteria that live there. That's another vital reason for helping your body to maintain the healthy balance of good and bad bacteria. When the delicate balance is lost, yeast may grow out of control. That overgrowth releases its own set of dangerous toxins or poisons, creating even more symptoms of IBS. It also causes fatigue, allergies, depression, chemical sensitivities and problems with immune function. (For more information on candida, please refer to my booklet *The Bible Cure Booklet for Candida and Yeast Infections.*)

Leaky Gut Syndrome

When the villi that line the small intestine have been damaged, tiny particles of undigested food, bacterial toxins and yeast toxins can pass freely into your bloodstream where they wreak all kinds

16

of havoc. The breakdown of this barrier is a condition known as *increased intestinal permeability* or *leaky gut syndrome.*

The foreign particles of food and other toxins in the blood may cause food allergies and sensitivities. Increased intestinal permeability commonly produces all of the symptoms of IBS, especially diarrhea after eating, bloating, gas and abdominal pain.

Conclusion

You can see that irritable bowel syndrome has many complicated components and causes. Your body was formed as the masterful work of a divine genius. Learning to properly care for God's amazing creation, your incredible body, shows that you have real wisdom and a genuine respect for your Creator.

The Bible says, "You made all the delicate, inner parts of my body and knit me together in my mother's womb. Thank you for making me so wonderfully complex! Your workmanship is marvelous—and how well I know it" (Ps. 139:13–14).

As you continue to unravel vital questions regarding IBS—its roots, causes and workings—you will gain the insight and godly wisdom you need to overcome this painful condition, not just temporarily, but permanently.

A BIBLE CURE PRAYER
FOR YOU

I pray that as you read this little booklet you will receive divine insight and fresh perspective that will bring this season of irritable bowel syndrome to an end. More importantly, I pray that God would impart fresh insight to you about Himself. His power to heal, His wisdom and His genuine love and compassion are yours right now. Let today mark the beginning of both physical and spiritual restoration. In Jesus' name, amen.

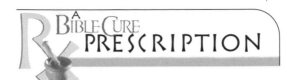

A BIBLE CURE PRESCRIPTION

Fill in the following blanks with your own name.

The Lord is _____ shepherd; _____ shall not want. He maketh _____ to lie down in green pastures: he leadeth me beside still waters. He restoreth _____ soul; he leadeth _____ in the paths of righteousness for his name's sake. Yea, though _____ walk through the valley of the shadow of death, I will fear no evil: for thou art with _____; thy rod and thy staff they comfort _____. Thou preparest a table before me in the presence of _____ enemies: thou anointest _____ head with oil; _____ cup runneth over. Surely goodness and mercy shall follow _____ all the days of _____ life: and _____ will dwell in the house of the Lord forever.
—ADAPTED FROM PSALM 23, KJV

Chapter 2

Restore With Nutrition

The Bible records historical accounts that show how stress and emotional turmoil can dramatically impact the normal functioning of your bowels. One biblical character, Job, endured a deeply stressful and difficult trial. Job personally describes how his stressful circumstances had affected his GI tract: "My bowels boiled, and rested not: the days of affliction prevented me" (Job 30:27, KJV).

IBS is often rooted in stress, emotional turmoil, difficult circumstances, poor diet and many other factors that can ravage your body's GI tract.

However, your wise Creator has provided much of what your body needs to combat naturally such physical distress. God's promise to you is complete restoration for your body, mind and spirit. The Bible says, "'For I will restore health to you and heal you of all your wounds,' says the LORD" (Jer. 30:17, NKJV).

A powerful avenue of this restoration for the physical body is through diet. One of God's wonderful works

> *Don't be troubled.*
> *You trust God, now*
> *trust in me.*
> —JOHN 14:1

as supernatural Creator was to provide the world with the foods that would perfectly suit your body's many and varied needs.

Nutritional Solutions for Healing

Your body, including your GI tract, was programmed by its Creator with unique powers to heal itself. You can do much to release your body's healing ability by exercising godly wisdom through the foods you choose to eat and those you choose to avoid for a short season.

Identifying Your Food Triggers

If you have irritable bowel syndrome, chances are good that you've already identified some food triggers that seem to make your symptoms worse. Here's a list of food triggers that negatively impact many individuals.

- Hot sauce
- Salsa
- Hot peppers
- Chili powder
- Barbecue sauce
- Curry sauce
- Garlic
- Caffeine

You can see that most of these food triggers are spicy foods, with the exception of caffeine. Most IBS sufferers cannot drink much coffee or other caffeinated beverages without causing IBS symptoms to flare up.

If you are experiencing IBS symptoms, don't drink more than one or two cups of coffee per day. If you have a cup in the morning, wait a few hours before pouring a second cup.

Other caffeinated beverages such as tea and sodas can have the same effect if you drink too much of them. The same rule of thumb applies to all caffeinated drinks. Limit the amount to two per day, and wait a couple of hours before having a second soda or cup of tea. You can enjoy all the caffeine-free herbal teas you want.

Suffering From Sorbitol?

If you are diabetic or do a lot of dieting, you may have noticed that some sugar-free foods tend to trigger IBS, too. Many times the reason for this is the sorbitol, an artificial sweetener. Sorbitol can be found in many sugar-free gums, diet choco-lates and sugar-free candies.

Some apple prod-ucts contain sorbitol. These include some varieties of apple juice and apple cider, as well as other canned fruits and fruit juices. Study the labels of all fruit and sugar-free products before purchasing them to see if they contain sorbitol.

> *Don't be afraid, for I am with you. Do not be dismayed, for I am your God. I will strengthen you. I will help you. I will uphold you with my righteous right hand.*
> —Isaiah 41:10

Believe it or not, even some toothpaste brands contain sorbitol. So, be sure to rinse your mouth out thoroughly after brushing, or select a natural brand of toothpaste that does not contain sorbitol.

Fructose Fury

Fructose is an extremely common IBS food trigger. If you have IBS, excessive fructose may cause bloat-ing, gas and diarrhea after you consume it. The reason for this is usually due to incomplete absorp-tion of the fructose.

Here are some foods with high concentrations of fructose that you'll want to avoid:

Cont'd

23

High in Fruitose

- Dried fruits (prunes, raisins, figs, dates)
- Honey
- Fruit juices
- Soft drinks
- Most candies

Grievous Gassy Foods

Some foods taste great, but they tend to create gas in your digestive tract. The reason is often a culprit called *raffinose,* which is a complex carbohydrate. Legumes or beans, tend to top this list. Cruciferous veggies cause problems for many people, too. Here's a list of food that can be gas generators for some individuals:

- Beans
- Peas
- Lentils
- Broccoli
- Brussels sprouts
- Cabbage
- Cauliflower
- Asparagus

Do any of these foods cause excessive gas? If so, add them to your list of offenders. The supplement Beano contains an enzyme that helps to eliminate gas caused by these foods.

Why Wheat Offends _Gluten_

Do wheat products cause symptoms of IBS in your body? If so, it may be that your body is allergic, sensitive or intolerant to wheat products. Or you may have a rarer condition called *celiac sprue.*

Celiac sprue results from an allergic reaction to gluten, which is a protein found mainly in wheat products. The allergic reaction in the gut damages the tiny villi lining the small intestine. When this happens, both fats and carbohydrates can no longer be properly absorbed by the body. Symptoms of celiac sprue are very similar to IBS, with one major exception. Celiac sprue will cause excessive diarrhea and lead to significant weight loss.

To treat celiac sprue you must eliminate all gluten-containing foods and products from your diet. Gluten-containing foods also include oats, barley and rye.

Frequent Fats

Overconsumption of fats is another extremely common trigger for irritable bowel syndrome. Usually the fats come from eating excessive amounts of fried food, margarine, butter, salad dressings, mayonnaise, cooking oils, cheeses, fatty cuts of meat and other high-fat foods.

What is your diet like? Do you eat fried foods every night and then wonder why you have irritable bowel syndrome? Even if your body was able to easily digest fats when you were a teenager, this may no longer be the case. Your body changes dramatically over the years, and your GI tract's ability to produce plenty of digestive juices to compensate for your over-indulgences diminishes with the passage of time.

Fats, especially bad fats, are very tough to digest. So, don't be surprised if your nutritional cure for IBS

> *Those who love your law have great peace and do not stumble.*
> —PSALM 119:165

requires you to take a hard look at the way you're presently eating. Once you've made the necessary dietary changes, you'll find that not only do you feel much better after you eat, but you also look better. Your clothes fit better as well.

Avoid Olestra

Olestra is a popular fat substitute that is calorie free and is being used in many low-calorie diet foods. A growing number of snack foods on the market contain Olestra, including potato chips, nachos and more.

The reason it is calorie-free is that the Olestra molecules, composed of sucrose (white sugar) and vegetable oil, are too large for your body to absorb, which causes them to pass through the GI tract and out of the body. That is why Olestra tends to cause a lot of gas, bloating, abdominal pain and diarrhea in many individuals.

Evade Alcohol

Do you enjoy an occasional drink, but find you experience a familiar and painful gut reaction when you do? The reason is that alcohol is another dietary trigger that you may need to avoid.

Alcohol irritates the lining of your GI tract and causes bloating, gas and diarrhea in many people with IBS.

Fiery Results From Fiber

Although fiber is essential for proper elimination and good health, soluble fiber can trigger painful IBS symptoms in some people. Many individuals who have IBS try to eat more fiber to combat it, not realizing that it may be making the symptoms even worse.

Soluble fiber found in oat bran, legumes, seeds (such as psyllium seed) and many over-the-counter fiber preparations can lead to increased fermentation in the GI tract, which creates more gas and bloating. Soluble fiber also may cause an overgrowth of normal intestinal bacteria.

A "No More Pain" Diet

Get a handle on your GI pain by starting a "No More Pain" elimination diet and journal. Many individuals with irritable bowel syndrome have food allergies, food sensitivities, food intolerances and food triggers. Therefore, an elimination diet can help you to identify what foods are causing you pain. I strongly encourage you to go on the following elimination diet to gain some insight into why your body is responding to normal eating experiences with pain, bloating, gas and other symptoms.

Here's How!

For starters, before you begin this essential elimination diet, purchase an inexpensive notebook and write the letters "N.M.P." (no more pain) on the front. You will need to keep an ongoing diary of your symptoms throughout the length of this diet. You can find a sample diary page as your Bible Cure prescription at the end of this chapter.

It is important to fill out the food diary at the end of each day and record any of the symptoms of IBS you experienced during the day.

In your diary, first write how painful your

symptoms were on a 1 to 10 scale, with 10 being the most severe and 1 being the least severe.

Next, record any possible foods that may have triggered your IBS. Refer to the lists in this booklet and any other lists of which you are aware.

Then, take a hard, long look at your eating habits. It may be that you've been stopping to grab a burger on your way to an evening meeting for years. The only difference is that now it's finally caught up with you. Also, think about the way you ate. Did you eat too fast? What about the time of day? Did you eat too late at night? Record all possible eating habit triggers in your journal, too.

> *But those who wait on the LORD will find new strength. They will fly high on wings like eagles. They will run and not grow weary. They will walk and not faint.*
> —ISAIAH 40:31

In addition to these natural causes of your discomfort, take a good, long look at the roots of your pain. Did you have an argument with your mate? Did your boss dump more work on you than you could possibly handle? Did your teenager leave the house on a date that has you worried? Record in your diary the stressful or worrisome situations that may have triggered your IBS pain.

29

Lining Up the Suspects

Now that you have your journal ready, you can get started with a diet that will help you find the culprit foods that are causing you pain.

The elimination diet

At first you must go on a very restricted diet that will not irritate your GI tract. After following the diet for a specified amount of time, you may begin to introduce the foods you suspect are irritating your gut as you record your body's reactions.

The *Janowitz Core Diet* was developed by renowned gastroenterologist Henry Janowitz, M.D. According to Dr. Janowitz, it's very rare for anyone to be sensitive to the foods on this very restricted diet.[1] The diet consists of the following:

- One meat, either chicken or lamb that is broiled, baked or roasted
- One starch, either rice or a baked potato (but only one)
- One canned fruit; Bartlett pears are recommended
- Bottled mineral water

Follow this strict diet for two to four weeks. After this period of time, introduce one food every other day and record your body's reactions. Introduce last the most likely trigger foods— foods high in fructose, caffeine, spicy foods, fatty foods, eggs, wheat and dairy and so forth.

If IBS symptoms occur, eliminate that particular trigger food from your diet. Wait until the symptoms of IBS are controlled before resuming your process of introducing new foods into your diet. Once the symptoms have resolved, begin introducing new foods every other day as before.

> *I will give you a new heart with new and right desires, and I will put a new spirit in you. I will take out your stony heart of sin and give you a new, obedient heart.*
> —EZEKIEL 36:26

Before long, you'll be well aware of which foods are triggering your painful IBS symptoms.

This diet works very well, but admittedly, it is extremely strict.

A BIBLE CURE HEALTH TIP

A Less Restrictive Diet

Another diet that is not so restricted includes making the right food choices from each food group.

Food	Avoid	Permitted
vegetables	legumes, beans, peas, lentils, broccoli, cabbage, Brussels sprouts and vegetables in a sauce	all others
fruit	citrus fruits (such as oranges, grapefruit, limes and lemons), canned fruits packed in sugar (avoid dried fruits and fruit juices)	all others
meat	sausage, processed meats, bacon, hamburgers, ham and all fried foods	lean beef, chicken and turkey breasts turkey breasts peeled off (Note: All meat should be baked, broiled or grilled—not fried. I recommend free-range meats.)
dairy products	all dairy, including milk, butter, cheese, ice cream, sour cream and yogurt	rice milk, soy milk, soy yogurt and almond milk
fish	all fried fish or breaded fish	any other fish

beverages	coffee, tea, sodas, fruit juices (especially orange juice), alcohol, tap water, grapefruit juice, lemonade	bottled or filtered water and herbal teas, like chamomile and peppermint tea
oils	all vegetable oils	small amounts of extra-virgin olive oil
starches	wheat, oats, rye, barley, corn	brown rice, white rice, rice cakes, millet bread, millet cereal, buckwheat, quinoa, rice cereal, spelt pasta

Avoid These Foods

While you're on the less-restricted diet described above, stay away from the following foods:

- Foods that contain yeast
- Vinegar
- Nuts
- Chocolate
- Honey
- Sugar (avoid sweets including candies,

cookies, doughnuts, cakes, pies)

After being on this restricted diet for two weeks, start introducing new foods every other day, as you would do with the elimination diet. If you begin experiencing symptoms of IBS after introducing a food item, eliminate that food and go back to the foods that did not cause your symptoms.

After two days, or when all symptoms pass, you may introduce other foods. Be sure to record in your food diary your symp-

> *He gives power to those who are tired and worn out; he offers strength to the weak.*
> —ISAIAH 40:29

toms, stress, the foods that trigger your symptoms and any eating patterns that you need to conquer. These include eating too fast, not chewing your food and other bad habits.

How You Eat and IBS

Most people with irritable bowel syndrome have poor eating patterns that make their condition much worse. Here's a description of the eating habits of a typical IBS patient. See if you can identify any of your eating habits in this scenario.

A typical IBS sufferer is notorious for eating on the run. She (or he) grabs a doughnut at 7-11 and gulps it down with hot coffee while fighting traffic on the freeway. She skips lunch, only to gulp down cookies at the snack machine when she takes a short break. She drinks a diet soda to wash them down in seconds, then runs breathlessly back to her desk.

Sound painfully familiar? Here's a list of the most common eating patterns shared by many IBS sufferers.

Eating when stressed

Many IBS sufferers eat under stressful circumstances or when they are tense and angry. This is terrible for your GI tract. If you are full of stress or frustration, release it. Bless your food, sit back, relax and get comfortable. Relaxing while eating is vital for helping your body digest and absorb your food properly.

Eating too fast

Some family dinner times look like a track event, the winner racing to the finish and leaving the table first.

If that sounds like your family, decide to slow down a little. Most people with IBS don't chew their food well enough to swallow, so they have to wash it down with a beverage. To insure proper digestion you should chew every bite of food at least twenty to thirty times.

You may have to make a real effort to slow down at meal times, since our whole culture is guilty of eating too quickly. You might need to pack your lunch the evening before so you won't have to wait in line at a restaurant. You will soon discover it's worth the effort, especially when your entire day feels more relaxed and you quit experiencing painful IBS symptoms.

When you eat too quickly you are also more prone to swallow a lot of air while eating, resulting in gas and bloating. To avoid these painful symptoms, sit down at every meal, relax and begin to make dining a peaceful experience.

Skipping meals

A lot of IBS sufferers skip meals throughout the day, only to eat massive quantities late in the evening for dinner. Never skip meals, and always allow about three to four hours between meals, as well as between your last meal and bedtime, so that your GI tract has a chance to digest your food.

Overeating

If you don't want to develop IBS symptoms, don't overeat. Decide before eating the meal how

36

much you are going to eat, and don't be tempted to go for seconds or eat sugary desserts. Also, learn to stop eating as soon as you are satisfied; never keep eating until you are stuffed.

Eating junk food

Avoid eating junk foods, fast foods and snack foods such as chips, French fries, pastries, doughnuts, cookies, pies, fried foods and candy bars. These foods tend to be much more difficult to digest, which can cause painful IBS symptoms.

Keeping these eating guidelines in mind every day will take you a long way in overcoming painful IBS symptoms. How you eat, as well as what you eat, is a major key in overcoming IBS.

> *So humble yourselves under the mighty power of God, and in his good time he will honor you. Give all your worries and cares to God, for he cares about what happens to you.*
> —1 PETER 5:6–7

Let's look now at what you eat that will help you overcome IBS.

Bowel Regularity

If you have been experiencing IBS, chances are you're well aware that regularity and your painful symptoms are closely related.

A major cause of IBS is simply an inconsistency in the speed at which your stools pass through your GI tract. If they pass too fast, you will develop diarrhea. But if they pass too slowly, you will become uncomfortably constipated.

Constipation is nothing more than passing a hard, small stool or having fewer than three bowel movements per week. If you do not drink enough water and eat enough fiber, or if you neglect your natural urge to go to the bathroom, you're likely to become constipated.

> *Those who have been ransomed by the LORD will return to Jerusalem, singing songs of everlasting joy. Sorrow and mourning will disappear, and they will be overcome with joy and gladness.*
> —ISAIAH 51:11

When the stool is small and hard from constipation, then the colon has to work much harder to eliminate it. The built-up pressure this causes can lead to spasms and cramps that create a great deal of pain.

Constipation has many causes. They include taking prescription medications such as narcotics and other pain medications, medications for hypertension, antacids, antihistamines and even iron tablets.

Other causes include inadequate water intake, lack of exercise and a lack of fiber in the diet.

"Eliminate the Negative"

Proper elimination through regular bowel movements is essential—your health and vitality depend on it! Without proper elimination, you cannot overcome irritable bowel syndrome.

If you are suffering from IBS, you may experience episodes of constipation alternating with episodes of diarrhea. This is quite common. If you have diarrhea often, your body may not be tolerating certain foods. The food elimination diet will help you discover what your food triggers are. Identifying food triggers, learning to relax and eating a high-fiber diet will help, along with some soothing herbs that we'll look at later.

Other keys to fighting constipation, as we have mentioned, are to drink at least two quarts of filtered water every day, exercise and never putting off your body's natural urge to have a bowel movement.

Your Fiber Needs

The best way to treat constipation is to eat a high-fiber diet. You may also take a fiber supplement.

You should be getting about 20 to 35 grams of fiber a day. Most people with IBS consume much less than that.

There is a danger, however, of taking too much fiber. Taking more than 35 grams of fiber a day can aggravate IBS symptoms. To help you avoid getting excessive amounts of fiber, it's important for you to be aware of the difference between soluble and insoluble fiber.

As I mentioned, getting between 20 and 35 grams of fiber on a daily basis is important. However, when you are consuming this much fiber, it's essential that you also drink enough water—no less than two quarts of filtered water daily. This is critically important.

Let's look at the different kinds of fiber available to you. There are six main types of fiber:

1. *Cellulose* is found in wheat bran and the peels of most fruits as well as the coating of most seeds. Cellulose fibers are insoluble fibers, which are excellent for those with IBS.
2. *Lignin* also is an insoluble fiber found in cereal grains and potato skins.

3. *Hemicellulose* is partly soluble and partly insoluble and is found in grains and wheat bran.

These first three types of fiber are best for you if you have irritable bowel syndrome since they are mostly insoluble fibers.

4. *Pectin* is a soluble fiber found in fruits.
5. *Gums* are found in vegetables, legumes, beans, lentils and oatmeal.
6. *Mucilage fiber* comes from seeds, such as psyllium seeds.

Here's a winning fiber ratio for your health: Try to get about two-thirds of your fiber in the form of insoluble fiber and about one-third as soluble fiber.

Fiber-Rich Foods

Many high-fiber foods, such as beans and other legumes, can trigger irritable bowel syndrome. If you do not have a food sensitivity to wheat, I recommend eating a high-fiber cereal every day, such as Fiber One, All Bran, Bran Buds or 100% Bran.

Start with a very small amount, about ¼ cup,

and gradually increase the amount to about ½ to 1 cup per day.

If you don't like the high-fiber cereals, then try a moderate-fiber cereal, which contains 4 to 5 grams of fiber per serving.

You may also increase your fiber by eating plenty of brown rice, eating the skins of potatoes and choosing whole-grain breads. Eat

> *You will keep in perfect peace all who trust in you, whose thoughts are fixed on you!*
> —Isaiah 26:3

plenty of fruits and vegetables, but be aware of your individual food triggers such as fructose, spicy foods, fatty foods or beans.

Although dried fruits such as raisins, figs, dates and prunes are great for fiber, they also are high in fructose and are common triggers for IBS. Therefore, you may find you have fewer symptoms without them.

In Conclusion

As you work through the dietary solutions given in this chapter, please remember that God is very concerned about your pain, whether it is great or relatively minor. Like a loving Father, one of His greatest pleasures is seeing you healthy, happy, genuinely fulfilled and blessedly restored from all of the ravages and assaults that you have suffered in life.

The restoration of your body, mind and spirit is extremely important to Him—so much so that He gave His own life to purchase your complete redemption. Never take His great love for you for granted!

A BIBLE CURE PRAYER
FOR YOU

Dear God, thank You for Your desire to restore and bring total healing to my body. Your love for me is truly amazing. Reveal that great love to me in a brand-new way. Bring restoration and total health to me as well—body, mind and spirit.

Thank You for the great price You paid on the cross so that I might walk in Your divine health. In Jesus' name, amen.

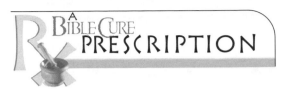

A BIBLE CURE PRESCRIPTION

Use this sample journal page to set up your N.M.P. journal.

N.M.P. JOURNAL

Foods I Have Eaten	Time Eaten

Amount of water I drank:

On a scale of 1 to 10, my symptoms were this painful:

My eating habits today were:

Chapter 3

Revive With Supplements

M ost of our lives are too full of cares, hurts, obstacles and disappointments. All of these emotions can release themselves right into our gut, resulting in IBS that becomes increasingly chronic. The prophet Jeremiah described his emotional distress and disappointment and how it affected his GI tract: "Mine eyes do fail with tears, my bowels are troubled" (Lam. 2:11, KJV).

Throughout the Bible, God's people express their need to be revived and restored emotionally, mentally, physically and spiritually. We read, "Wilt thou not revive us again: that thy people may rejoice in thee? Shew us thy mercy, O LORD, and grant us thy salvation" (Ps. 85:6–7, KJV).

Chances are that you may need reviving,

renewing and restoring just as much, if not more, than do these great men of the Bible. Your restoration will begin as you understand God's deep desire to see you well, healed, whole and joyful, not just spiritually, but physically, mentally and emotionally, too.

To begin the healing process and physical renewal that God desires for you, you must target one of the places where stress can create the most havoc—your GI tract. You can do this with the help of powerful supplements that will go right to work to soothe and heal the damage.

Supplements for IBS

Let's look at some supplements that are vital for your recovery.

Good bacteria

When you suffer with IBS, supplementing your body's own good bacteria is essential. It may be hard to believe that more than four hundred different kinds of bacteria are living in your colon right now. These friendly bacteria are necessary to health.

The most important friendly bacteria are the lactobacillus acidophilus and bifidobacterium. To increase their presence in your digestive tract, you can take them as supplements.

I recommend about 3 billion colony-forming units of L-acidophilus and bifidobacterium once or twice a day. Biodophilus from Biotics is an excellent supplement that contains beneficial bacteria. To order this product call 800-874-7318.

FOS

FOS (fructo-oligosaccharides) are sugars that promote the growth of good bacteria. I usually recommend about 2000 milligrams of FOS daily. Occasionally some patients with IBS do not tolerate this supplement. Biodophilus also contains FOS.

Homeostatic soil organisms

This supplement is a form of Probiotics under the name *Primal Defense.* Primal Defense contains fifteen strains of good bacteria including lactobacillus acidophilus, bifidobacterium bifidis, lactobacillus plantarum and so forth. This is the best Probiotics supplement that I have used.

I recommend two tablets of Primal Defense twice a day on an empty stomach. To order Primal Defense call 800-580-PLUS.

Digestive enzymes

IBS sufferers usually need to take a digestive enzyme that supplies adequate amounts of the following enzymes: protease, lipase, amylase. Choose a tablet instead of a capsule because some IBS patients are sensitive to capsules.

Bio-6-Plus from Biotics or Divine Health Vegetarian Enzyme are good digestive enzyme supplements. I recommend one to two tablets with each meal. Call Biotics at 800-874-7318 to order Bio-6-Plus and 407-331-7007 to order the latter.

Moducare

Moducare is a phytonutrient of plant sterols and sterolins (plant oils) that has helped many patients with IBS. Symptoms caused by food triggers can be reduced or eliminated. Elevated cortisol levels caused by excessive stress will also be balanced. I recommend two tablets (veggie caps) three times a day for the first week one hour before meals, and one tablet three times a day thereafter. To order this product call 407-331-7007.

Peppermint oil

Peppermint oil may be effective for decreasing colon spasms, diarrhea and other IBS symptoms. However, peppermint oil must be taken in enteric-coated tablets. Otherwise, the volatile compounds in the peppermint oil will be absorbed before they can reach the lower GI tract.

Take one to two enteric-coated tablets between meals.

Chamomile tea

This soothing relaxant is used often for cramping abdominal pain. However, if you are allergic to ragweed it may cause an allergic reaction.

Brew chamomile tea in a covered container and use as often as you need for abdominal pain.

Slippery elm

Slippery elm is an herb used to soothe irritated tissues, such as irritation in the small or large bowel. Slippery elm can be consumed as tea or taken in its herbal form. Just avoid gelatin capsules since these can aggravate IBS.

You may take slippery elm lozenges three times per day.

Glutamine

When treating IBS, it's extremely important to repair the lining of the small intestine or heal the leaky gut. The amino acid glutamine is one of the most important supplements for repairing the GI tract.

Take 500 milligrams to 1000 milligrams thirty minutes before meals three times a day. Take a caplet or powder form rather than a capsule.

Excess stress, anxiety or depression may also be associated with IBS. Let's look at some supplements that can help.

Supplements for depression

If you are battling depression, select one supplement from the following list:

- 5-HTP (50 mg. three times per day)
- SAM-e (200 to 400 mg. two times per day on an empty stomach)
- St. John's Wort (300 mg. three times per day)

Don't take any of these supplements if you are taking a prescription antidepressant medicine. Please refer to my booklet *The Bible Cure for Depression and Anxiety.*

Supplement for anxiety and stress

An excellent supplement for anxiety and stress is Kava. This supplement is not addictive like medications such as Xanax and Valium. It does not impair mental functioning, and it works well for both anxiety and depression. Take 45 to 90 milligrams of Kava three times per day. You may also take Kava as an herbal tincture or as a tea.

Overcoming Constipation

IBS sufferers tend to spend much of their time dealing with either constipation or diarrhea or both at different times. Dealing with constipation in a natural, healthy way will help.

Many people are dependent upon laxatives to have a bowel movement. If you are among them, it is essential to restore your body to normal functioning. Avoid all stimulant laxatives, including herbal laxatives such as "senna" and "cascara sagrada." These remedies stimulate the bowel muscles to contract, which may actually worsen symptoms of IBS.

He comforts us in all our troubles so that we can comfort others. When others are troubled, we will be able to give them the same comfort God has given us.
—2 CORINTHIANS 1:4

The safest laxatives are the bulk-forming varieties of various kinds of fiber.

Fantastic Fiber

Natural wheat bran provides the best way to get the fiber your body needs. It is also called Miller's bran or Baker's bran, and it looks like sawdust. Start by taking 1 tablespoon daily and gradually increase the amount to 1 tablespoon two times per day. Eventually, work up to 2 tablespoons two times per day.

You can mix this fiber with hot cereal, sprinkle it over other cereals or add it to baked goods or to a smoothie. As long as one does not have any kind of wheat intolerance, this fiber is a good choice. Most individuals with IBS tolerate it well.

If you have a wheat sensitivity, you need to avoid these types of fiber. Here is a list of other good types of fiber that you may select:

1. *Methylcellulose.* The brand Citrucel contains this type of fiber. This brand typically contains sucrose or NutraSweet. Locate a brand without sucrose or NutraSweet at your favorite health food store.

2. *Rice bran.* This is a wonderful source of fiber for those with a sensitive GI tract. I recommend starting with 1 tablespoon of rice bran a day, gradually increasing the dosage to 2 tablespoons two times per day. Ultra fiber from Metagenics is an excellent rice bran fiber. Call 800-647-6100

for information on obtaining this product.

3. *The husks of psyllium seeds.* You can find this fiber source in Metamucil, Perdiem Fiber and many other over-the-counter preparations. They are an excellent source of both insoluble and soluble fiber. (Avoid brands that contain sugar or NutraSweet.) Start introducing this fiber into your diet slowly by taking only 1 teaspoon a day. Gradually increase the amount to 1 tablespoon two times a day.

4. *Calcium polycarbophil.* This is a synthetic fiber that cannot be fermented by bacteria. FiberCon is an example of it. Take it according to the package directions.

Supplements will go right to work supporting, relaxing and soothing your GI tract, however gelatin capsules and caplets may aggravate IBS in some patients; if so, they should be avoided.

In Conclusion

Your total restoration includes your body, mind

and spirit. Understanding God's deep desire for your wholeness and healing is a key to unlocking the power of His love in your life.

God is more than a healer. He is *your* healer who loves you with a depth of love that your mind is not big enough to even imagine. He is committed to you, and He suffered on the cross so that you could be whole. Never doubt His great love for you.

A BIBLE-CURE PRAYER
FOR YOU

Dear Lord, I pray that You might open up the eyes of this one reading this booklet. Reveal Your great love and awesome power to heal, restore and revive. I'm thankful that it is not Your desire that anyone should suffer. As a matter of fact, You died on the cross so that we might be saved and healed. Restore this precious individual's body to the place of perfect health. In Jesus' name, amen.

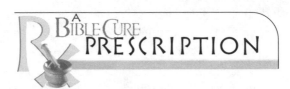

Circle the supplements you take daily and underline those you plan to begin taking.

Good bacteria	Glutamine
FOS	5-HTP
Digestive enzymes	St. John's Wort
Peppermint oil	Sam-e
Chamomile tea	Kava
Slippery elm	Moducare

How do you plan to address your body's need for fiber?

_____

_____

_____

Write a prayer asking God to reveal His great love for you in an entirely new way.

_____

_____

_____

Chapter 4

Reinvigorate With Exercise

Even if you feel worn out and depleted because of stress and the physical symptoms of IBS, God has good news for you. He promises to strengthen and reinvigorate your life. The Bible says, "He gives power to those who are tired and worn out; he offers strength to the weak" (Isa. 40:29).

You can discover a brand-new you in God, a you who radiates health, life and peace. Another key to obtaining the vision of all that God intends for you is the strength that your body can receive through exercise and relaxation.

Discovering Quietness

As a society, we've lost our love for quiet places,

times and spaces. Think for a moment about your life. You get up, turn the radio or television on, shout over the noise of your children and rush out into traffic. Horns honk and frustrations build as you race into work to face a mountain of pressure.

Although you may be accustomed to this kind of stress-filled lifestyle, it still places an enormous toll upon the health of your body and mind. Releasing some of that daily stress through regular exercises and relaxation techniques can work wonders for you. Some are very simple to do anytime.

Devote Yourself to Deep Breathing

Here are a few deep breathing techniques that are easy to do and can change your life.

When you are stressed, your breathing tends to become rapid and shallow. The most relaxed breathing is slow, abdomen-centered breathing from the diaphragm, which is far healthier for your body. Do this exercise when you sense that your breathing is becoming stressed.

1. Find a quiet place and sit or lie down in a comfortable position. Close your eyes and place one hand on your

chest and the other hand on your abdomen. Determine where your breathing is coming from. Is it coming from your chest or abdomen? Abdominal breathing has a calming effect on the body. However, most people are chest breathers.

2. Correct your shallow, stress-filled breathing by lying on your back. Place a book on your lower abdomen below your navel. As you breathe in, the book should rise. As you breathe out, it should sink.

3. Breathe in deeply and slowly. Pause and relax.

4. Repeat until you begin to feel calmer and more relaxed.

Deep muscle relaxation exercises can release your body, muscles and internal organs (especially your GI tract) from the grip of destructive stress.

The following three-minute relaxation routine can be a lifesaver in a tense situation.

1. Concentrate on relaxing using a cue word, such as *God's peace* or *God's love*. Listen to your own breathing,

59

and take in one deep breath and hold it.

2. While you are holding your breath, tense up a group of muscles, such as the muscles in your face, legs or arms.

3. As you release your breath, relax the tense muscle group. Feel all your tension slip away. Drop your shoulders down and rotate them in a circle.

4. Repeat.

You can do this relaxation exercise anywhere Relaxation training reduces anxiety and stress, and it decreases heart disease and high blood pressure as well.[1]

Progressive Muscle Relaxation

This relaxation exercise can relax your entire body in about twenty minutes.

1. Sit or lie down quietly in a comfortable position away from noise or distractions.

2. Tense and tighten your muscles in each of the following muscle groups beginning at your head. Tense each

body part for five seconds, and then slowly release the tension as you focus on the body part. This needs to be repeated twice for each muscle group.

- Forehead and top of head—raise eyebrows
- Jaw—clench teeth
- Neck—pull chin forward onto your chest and then push your head back
- Shoulders and trapezoid muscles—lift shoulders
- Back—pull back shoulder blades
- Arms—flex biceps
- Abdomen—tighten abdomen
- Buttocks—squeeze and tighten buttocks
- Thighs—flex thighs
- Calves—flex and point toes up or down

As you learn to slowly release the tension in your muscles, you will actually be teaching your body how to relax.

Get Hooked on Regular Exercise

Aerobic exercise also helps to calm your body as well as your mind by releasing tension. Regular aerobic exercise doesn't have to be a chore; it can be a lot of fun. One of the best exercises to perform is brisk walking. But the best exercise for you is the one you will enjoy doing on a regular basis, perhaps with a friend or family member. Refer to my booklet *The Bible Cure Booklet on Stress* for a detailed exercise program.

Regular exercise improves heart health, lung function, circulation and blood pressure. It reduces fat and lowers cholesterol. Regular exercise relaxes your muscles, reduces stress and decreases fatigue. As you exercise, your body also releases endorphins, which are natural antidepressants that make you feel better, relieve pain and give you a renewed sense of well-being.

So, to boost your self-image, build your confidence and increase your energy, determine to start exercising twenty minutes a day for at least three days per week.

In Conclusion

Renewed vigor, excitement, strength and joy are yours in God. Total restoration is His plan for your life—and He will accomplish His plan when we are willing for it. The Bible says, "But those who wait on the LORD will find new strength. They will fly high on wings like eagles. They will run and not grow weary. They will walk and not faint" (Isa. 40:31).

God has truly wonderful things ahead for you—great times and blessed experiences in Him that you cannot even imagine. So go ahead. Get going! Begin running to not grow weary, and walking to not faint. Before long, I trust that truly you will be flying high with wings like an eagle!

A BIBLE CURE PRAYER
FOR YOU

Dear God, I pray that You give me the discipline and help that I need to begin exercising my body. I thank You that Your deep desire for me is that I would be whole and healthy in my body, mind and spirit. I receive Your great and wonderful love for me, although I really don't understand it. Give me the grace to look to You every day for the help I need. Amen.

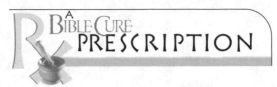

A BIBLE CURE PRESCRIPTION

Do you exercise rarely, occasionally or regularly?

_____

What hindrances or obstacles keep you from exercising?

_____

_____

Outline a strategy for overcoming these obstacles using prayer and the Word of God as guides.

_____

_____

_____

Write a prayer asking God for His help in maintaining a regular exercise routine.

_____

_____

_____

Chapter 5

Renew With God's Word

We have seen the dramatic effect that stressful circumstances and emotional turmoil can have in causing IBS. When war and turmoil came to ancient Israel, the prophet Jeremiah cried, "My bowels, my bowels! I am pained at my very heart; my heart maketh a noise in me; I cannot hold my peace, because thou hast heard, O my soul, the sound of the trumpet, the alarm of war" (Jer. 4:19, KJV). Jeremiah's circumstances shook him to the very core, and he cried out with the pain of his physical symptoms as they attacked his gut.

Even if you are facing impossible circumstances in your life that are creating seemingly insurmountable stress, physical and emotional distress is not God's will for you. He desires to completely revive and restore you—body, mind and spirit. Understanding how your reactions to stress affect you and learning biblical keys to renewing your mind through God's Word will help you to rise above painful situations.

Your Mind-Gut Connection

To understand the relationship between IBS, your emotions and the stress with which you cope every day it's vital to understand your mind-gut connection.

The human body is an amazing creation; it is more complex than we realize. Your mind and body are not as disconnected as we've been led to believe. A thought that overwhelms your emotions can directly impact your GI tract.

Has this ever happened to you? Like the ancient prophet Jeremiah, have you experienced panic or fear that immediately upset your digestion?

Your thoughts can upset the GI tract, leading to increased contractions.

Our minds are sensitive to subtle suggestions. The memory of previous painful GI experiences can create a perception that a GI event is about to occur when what is really happening is very normal. In fact, it's possible for previous painful episodes to cause a person to become very focused on his or her GI tract, immediately noticing and constantly monitoring unusual feelings.

Such intense focus can set up an individual to perceive relatively minor sensations as indications of an impending problem. In truth, some of these minor sensations are common and have no clinical significance.

> *I am convinced that nothing can ever separate us from his love. Nothing in all creation will ever be able to separate us from the love of God that is revealed in Christ Jesus our Lord.*
> —ROMANS 8:38–39

Individuals who aren't anticipating GI trouble wouldn't notice them.

I'm *not* suggesting that your experience of pain is merely in your head. It is very real pain caused by very real physical factors. Understanding some of those factors will be helpful to relieve some of your anxiety when they occur.

Adrenaline and Stress Attacks

When something extremely stressful happens, the body produces adrenaline. When something similar happens, your body holds within it a memory of the former event, which triggers another release of adrenaline similar to the first one. So, adrenaline is released regardless of the actual physical circumstances.

Adrenaline is an extremely powerful chemical that can cause diarrhea or abdominal cramps. Though this is normally recognized as a minor episode for most, it is not so for IBS sufferers. That's because those with irritable bowel syndrome tend to interpret these symptoms as something wrong happening in their bodies.

Now a vicious cycle is created because early perceived signs of IBS actually cause more stress and anxiety, which causes more symptoms of IBS.

This is the mind-gut connection, which is at the root of much IBS pain and ongoing distress.

Over the Edge of Stress

When an individual is at the point at which even minor stress can trigger painful physical responses, he or she is teetering near the edge. The situation can get even worse, however. When the GI tract is able to upset the mind to the point of leading to anxiety, depression or even substance abuse, then he or she has developed a *somatoform disorder.*

Somatoform disorder occurs when an individual becomes overly focused on his or her body and becomes unusually aware and keenly sensitive to sensations that have no real significance. Although this can happen to all IBS sufferers, it is considered a disorder when it becomes severe enough to interfere with day-to-day living.

If your doctor is unable to diagnose a specific illness, he or she generally concludes that it's a somatoform disorder. IBS is often rooted in a somatoform disorder. However, other emotional disorders are commonly seen with IBS, such as generalized anxiety disorder, depression and even substance abuse. For more information concerning anxiety and depression, please refer to my booklet *The Bible Cure Booklet for Depression and Anxiety.*

Understanding the Types of Stress

Stress has many faces, for many types of stress exist. Major life events create one type of stress. These include the death of a loved one, a divorce, getting married, an accident, the loss of a job, a move and much more. (See the Holmes Ray scale in the *The Bible Cure for Stress.*)

In addition, modern life is filled with many minor stresses. These include arguments with your spouse or friends, your children's discipline problems, traffic jams, deadlines, an irritating boss, the demands of raising small children, financial pressures and more.

Still, we can easily turn our minor stress into major stress through the process of our own perceptions and reactions. This adds to our stress level and can dramatically aggravate irritable bowel syndrome.

Silencing Stressful Reactions

If we're honest with ourselves, we'll admit that the way we perceive much of our personal stress is a result of our individual disposition and personality makeup. One individual can undergo extremely stressful circumstances and remain as cool as a cucumber, while another with a different personality type experiences extreme stress caused by the most minor provocations.

Like it or not, your level of stress is going to be greatly influenced by your belief system. To change your stress level you must be willing to take a hard look at your beliefs, perceptions and reactions.

If you're like many people, you may feel that you don't have a particularly individualized system of beliefs and reactions. But you do. Changing your perception of stressful situations will launch you into a brand-new outlook on life that can bring you great freedom.

To control stress, you must learn to see stressful situations as they are—nothing more than daily nuisances and hassles. Begin developing skills to help you cope with the constant bombardment of daily stresses. Learn to both calm your mind and relax your body.

Identifying Self-Cursing

Our faulty perception of our own worth also causes stress. Many of us don't need others or even the devil to attack our self-esteem. We do a great job of tearing ourselves down. You may well be cursing yourself all day long. That may sound shocking, so let me explain.

Negative self-talk is a way that we curse and tear ourselves down. If we were to isolate our negative thoughts about ourselves, they might sound something like the following:

- "Boy, am I stupid!"
- "What is the matter with me?"
- "I feel so fat and ugly."

Are you getting the picture? Most of us would never say such horrible things to another person.

71

We would consider it cruel to do so. But we speak such awful things to ourselves often without a second thought. Have you ever considered that speaking to yourself in such a fashion offends your Creator? It absolutely does!

Negative self-talk produces a self-cursing that can undermine all that you are. Such unkind words create an internal belief system about yourself that can destroy your confidence, defeat your dreams and bring sickness upon you. Negative self-talk robs you of the blessings God wants to place upon your life.

Stop It!

It's extremely important to identify and eliminate undermining negative self-talk. To change your perceptions of yourself, you must first identify your self-talk. Whether you realize it or not, a continual dialogue of words and emotions goes on in your head. Here's how to really examine what you're saying to yourself:

1. Carry a journal or small, hand-held recorder around with you for about a month.
2. As you go through your daily life,

record the thoughts that spontaneously come into your head. Although this may feel awkward at first, it's important.

3. As you record your self-talk, draw a dash and record briefly where the self-talk is taking place. For instance: "I hate being late!"—rush-hour traffic jam.

4. At the end of the month, review what you've written or recorded.

5. Make a list of all the negative comments you've made about yourself.

6. Consider how you would feel if your spouse or best friend said those things to you.

7. List the negative statements that occur most often.

Neutralizing the Power of Self-Curses

Write down each destructive self-thought and write a corresponding scripture beside it. This important exercise requires a good concordance and several prayerful hours to make it work. Here's an example:

- *Negative self-thought:* "I hate the way I

look. I feel so fat!"—getting dressed for a social occasion.

- *Corresponding scripture:* "And God saw everything that he had made, and, behold, it was very good" (Gen. 1:31, KJV).

Writing the Word on Your Heart

God desires that His Word be written upon the tablets of our hearts. Hebrews 8:10 says, "This is the new covenant I will make with the house of Israel on that day, says the Lord. I will put my laws in their minds so they will understand them, and I will write them on their hearts."

The Word of God has the ability to destroy the root of those negative self-curses and replace them with godly blessings promised in His Word.

Write down the various scriptures you have discovered through your prayerful search on 3- x 5-inch index cards, and carry them

> *For the law was given through Moses; God's unfailing love and faithfulness came through Jesus Christ.*
> —JOHN 1:17

with you wherever you go. Before long you'll discover the power of these words to extinguish the fiery curses of negativity that have found a place in your mind and spirit.

Getting a Grip on Stress

If your life is filled with stress, you may need to begin making some changes—for your health's sake.

Here's how:

1. List all of the things in your life that are creating stress for you.
2. Take a hard look at what items can be eliminated or dealt with in a different manner.
3. Write down a list of your goals.
4. Analyze your list by asking the following question: Which goals are truly my own goals as a result of prayer, and which ones are goals placed upon me by someone else (such as mother, wife, friends, etc.)?
5. Cut your stress list in half by eliminating the heavy weight of burdens you were never intended to carry.

Your Deadline Dilemma

You will never get control over your stress if you do not take strong steps to control your day, your diet and your deadlines. Take a careful—and prayerful—look at your deadlines. Do you wait too long to leave for work? Do you procrastinate performing important tasks?

With some forethought, you can develop some new strategies to reduce your deadline stress. Which deadlines can you renegotiate? In what ways can you become more organized to speed your projects along?

Forgive, Forget and Apologize

The final key to renew-ing your mind and your life through God's Word is implementing the power of forgive-

> *He heals the broken-hearted, binding up their wounds.*
> —PSALM 147:3

ness. The Bible says, "Do not judge, and you will not be judged. Do not condemn, and you will not be condemned. Forgive, and you will be forgiven" (Luke 6:37, NIV).

Holding a grudge requires a great deal of energy and robs you of your joy. Unforgiveness is a deadly emotion that can cause disease in your body, mind and spirit. It is vital to learn to release people from unforgiveness. The following exercise can be helpful:

- Pull a chair up to the center of your living

room, bedroom or study.
- Now, prayerfully pretend to place the individual who wronged you on that chair.
- Symbolically write that person's name on a card and lay the card on the chair.
- Now, speak aloud to that invisible person.
- Recite in detail what he (or she) did that wounded you.
- Tell him how he made you feel when he wronged you.
- Explain why it hurt.
- Tell him why you feel angry.
- Now, finally, announce to the individual that you are forgiving him or her.
- You don't need to justify your forgiveness. Simply recite the Word of God regarding forgiveness and declare that you are obeying it. You may feel like crying. If so, go ahead and cry. You may feel like shouting, so feel free to do so. What's important is that you forgive.
- Announce aloud that this person is free from the bondage of your anger, resentment and bitterness. Say, "I release you, _____; you are free."
- Write the word *forgiven* on the card over the individual's name.

- Finally, if you are able, hold the card up to heaven and ask God to bless this person. Just as Christ said on the cross, pray, "Father, forgive _____ for he/she didn't know what he/she was doing."

Wipe Clean Your Slate

Pray and ask God if there are others whom you've neglected to forgive whose names you cannot remember. Ask God to search your heart and wipe it clean of any bitterness, anger, resentment or unforgiveness. In addition, in some situations it is important to go and attempt to repair or build a relationship bridge with that individual. Ask God in prayer if He desires it in your situation.

Love Says I'm Sorry

Is there someone who needs to pretend to place you on a chair and speak words of forgiveness over you? If you're honest with yourself, you may realize that there are several people who feel wronged by you.

If you have wronged anyone in any way, apologize to that person as an expression of God's love through you. As you do, you'll be reinvigorated with a fresh sense of joy that comes from touching God's heart.

A BIBLE CURE PRAYER
FOR YOU

Dear God, I thank You for Your love and healing power to restore even the most needy and broken places in our lives. I pray that You touch this precious reader with the power of Your wonderful Spirit. Renew this one with the dynamic truth of Your wonderful Word. Restore and refresh with Your tender mercies and gentle lovingkindness. Revive this one You love with Your abundant grace. In Jesus' name, amen.

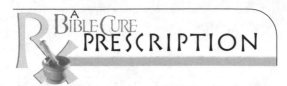

A BIBLE CURE PRESCRIPTION

List some of the negative self-talk and self-cursing statements that you've heard yourself make.

_____

_____

Describe the circumstances surrounding this self-talk.

_____

_____

What corresponding scriptures will you use to renew your mind and heart regarding these destructive self-statements?

_____

_____

Write a prayer thanking God for creating you—imperfections and all!

_____

_____

List those individuals you need to forgive. Start by forgiving yourself of any shortcomings, negative self-talk, etc.

————————————————————

————————————————————

List those individuals to whom you need to apologize.

————————————————————

————————————————————

Write a prayer thanking God for His wonderful love for you. Thank Him for forgiving you of all of your sins.

————————————————————

————————————————————

A PERSONAL NOTE

From Don and Mary Colbert

God desires to heal you of disease. His Word is full of promises that confirm His love for you and His desire to give you His abundant life. His desire includes more than physical health for you; He wants to make you whole in your mind and spirit as well through a personal relationship with His Son, Jesus Christ.

If you haven't met my best friend, Jesus, I would like to take this opportunity to introduce Him to you. It is very simple.

If you are ready to let Him come into your heart and become your best friend, just bow your head and sincerely pray this prayer from your heart:

Lord Jesus, I want to know You as my Savior and Lord. I believe You are the Son of God and that You died for my sins. I also believe You were raised from the dead and now sit at the right hand of the Father praying for me. I ask You to forgive me for my sins and change my heart so that I can be Your child and live with You eternally.

Thank You for Your peace. Help me to
walk with You so that I can begin to know
You as my best friend and my Lord. Amen.

If you have prayed this prayer, we rejoice
with you in your decision and your new relationship with Jesus. Please contact us at
pray4me@strang.com so that we can send you
some materials that will help you become estab-
lished in your relationship with the Lord. You
have just made the most important decision of
your life. We look forward to hearing from you.

Notes

CHAPTER 2
RESTORE WITH NUTRITION

1. Henry Janowitz, M.D., *Your Gut Feelings* (New York: Random House, 1994).

CHAPTER 4
REINVIGORATE WITH EXERCISE

1. Trevor Powell, *Free Yourself From Harmful Stress* (New York: DJ Publishing, 1997), 128.

Don Colbert, M.D., was born in Tupelo, Mississippi. He attended Oral Roberts School of Medicine in Tulsa, Oklahoma, where he received a bachelor of science degree in biology in addition to his degree in medicine. Dr. Colbert completed his internship and residency with Florida Hospital in Orlando, Florida. He is board certified in family practice and has received extensive training in nutritional medicine.

If you would like more
information about natural and
divine healing, or information about
Divine Health Nutritional Products®,
you may contact
Dr. Colbert at:

DR. DON COLBERT

1908 Boothe Circle
Longwood, FL 32750
Telephone: 407-331-7007
(For ordering products only)

Dr. Colbert's website is
www.drcolbert.com.

Disclaimer: Dr. Colbert and the staff of Divine Health Wellness Center are prohibited from addressing a patient's medical condition by phone, facsimile or e-mail. Please refer questions related to your medical condition to your own primary care physician.

Pick up these other Siloam Press
books by Dr. Colbert:

Toxic Relief

Walking in Divine Health

What You Don't Know May Be Killing You

The Bible Cure® Booklet Series

The Bible Cure for ADD and Hyperactivity
The Bible Cure for Allergies
The Bible Cure for Arthritis
The Bible Cure for Back Pain
The Bible Cure for Cancer
The Bible Cure for Candida and Yeast Infection
The Bible Cure for Chronic Fatigue and Fibromyalgia
The Bible Cure for Depression and Anxiety
The Bible Cure for Diabetes
The Bible Cure for Headaches
The Bible Cure for Heart Disease
The Bible Cure for Heartburn and Indigestion
The Bible Cure for Hepatitis and Hepatitis C
The Bible Cure for High Blood Pressure
The Bible Cure for Irritable Bowel Syndrome
The Bible Cure for Memory Loss
The Bible Cure for Menopause
The Bible Cure for Osteoporosis
The Bible Cure for PMS and Mood Swings
The Bible Cure for Prostate Disorders
The Bible Cure for Skin Disorders
The Bible Cure for Sleep Disorders
The Bible Cure for Stress
The Bible Cure for Weight Loss and Muscle Gain

SILOAM PRESS
A part of Strang Communications Company
600 Rinehart Road
Lake Mary, FL 32746
(800) 599-5750